JUICING RECIPES FOR GUT HEALTH

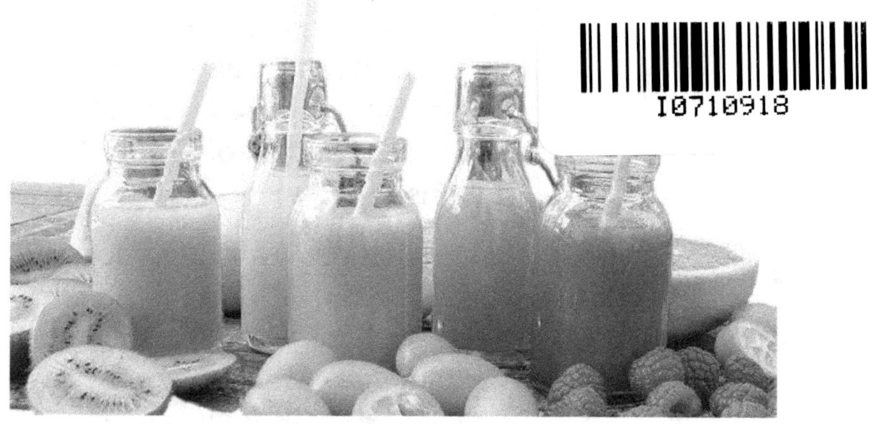

Delicious and Nutritious Recipes for a
Healthy Digestive System

Wilbert M. Jensen

TABLE OF CONTENT

INTRODUCTION OF JUICING RECIPES FOR GUT HEALTH

Godwin was always interested in finding natural ways to improve his health. So when he started experiencing digestive issues, he began to research the best ways to heal his gut. That's when he stumbled upon juicing.

He learned that juicing fruits and vegetables was a great way to get all the nutrients his body needed to heal his gut. With a juicer in hand, he set out to find the best juicing recipes for gut health.

Godwin experimented with different combinations of fruits and vegetables until he found the perfect recipe. He found that mixing kale, spinach, cucumber, celery, ginger, and apple together in a juicer created a delicious and nutritious drink that was perfect for his gut.

He began to drink this juice every morning, and he noticed a significant improvement in his gut health. He no longer experienced bloating or discomfort, and he had more energy throughout the day.

Godwin was so impressed with the power of juicing that he started to share his recipes with his friends and family. He even started a blog to share his juicing recipes with people around the world.

Thanks to his dedication to juicing and his passion for natural health remedies, Godwin became an expert in juicing for gut health. He continued to explore new combinations of fruits and vegetables to create even more delicious and healthy recipes.

In the end, Godwin's journey to heal his gut led him to discover a whole new way of life. By embracing the power of natural remedies like juicing, he was able to transform his health and inspire others to do the same.

In recent years, there has been a growing interest in juicing as a natural way to improve gut health. Juicing involves extracting the liquid from fruits and vegetables, which allows the body to easily absorb all the nutrients they contain.

By incorporating juicing into your daily routine, you can help support the health of your gut, which plays a crucial role in overall health and wellbeing. With the right combination of fruits and vegetables, you can create delicious and nutritious juices that are specifically designed to promote gut health.

Whether you're looking to heal digestive issues or simply maintain a healthy gut, juicing is a powerful tool that can help you achieve your goals. In this article, we will explore some of the best juicing recipes for gut health and explain how they can benefit your body.

CHAPTER 1

Overview of Juicing for Gut Health

Juicing has gained popularity as a natural remedy for improving gut health in recent years. Our gut, also known as the gastrointestinal tract, is responsible for the digestion and absorption of nutrients from the food we eat.

The health of our gut is closely linked to our overall wellbeing, with gut health playing a critical role in maintaining a healthy immune system, regulating metabolism, and improving mental health.

Juicing involves extracting the liquid from fruits and vegetables, which is believed to provide a concentrated source of nutrients that can be easily absorbed by the body. The nutrients found in fruits and vegetables, such as vitamins, minerals, and antioxidants, are essential for maintaining a healthy gut.

Juicing for gut health is a great way to increase the intake of nutrients that are known to support the health of the digestive system. The nutrients found in fruits and vegetables help to nourish the cells that line the gut and support the growth of beneficial gut bacteria, which are critical for optimal digestive health.

Some of the best fruits and vegetables for juicing for gut health include:

Leafy Greens - Kale, spinach, and collard greens are rich in vitamins and minerals that support digestive health.

Cruciferous Vegetables - Broccoli, cauliflower, and cabbage are rich in sulfur-containing compounds that support detoxification and improve digestion.

Ginger - Ginger is a powerful anti-inflammatory that can help to soothe the digestive system and reduce inflammation in the gut.

Berries - Berries are rich in antioxidants and fiber, which support healthy digestion and regulate bowel movements.

By incorporating these fruits and vegetables into your juicing routine, you can support the health of your gut and promote optimal digestive function.

In conclusion, juicing for gut health is a simple and effective way to improve your overall health and wellbeing. By incorporating nutrient-rich fruits and vegetables into your daily routine, you can support the health of your gut and improve your digestive function. With the right combination of ingredients, you can create delicious and nutritious juices that are specifically designed to promote gut health. So why not give it a try and see how juicing can benefit your gut health and overall wellbeing!

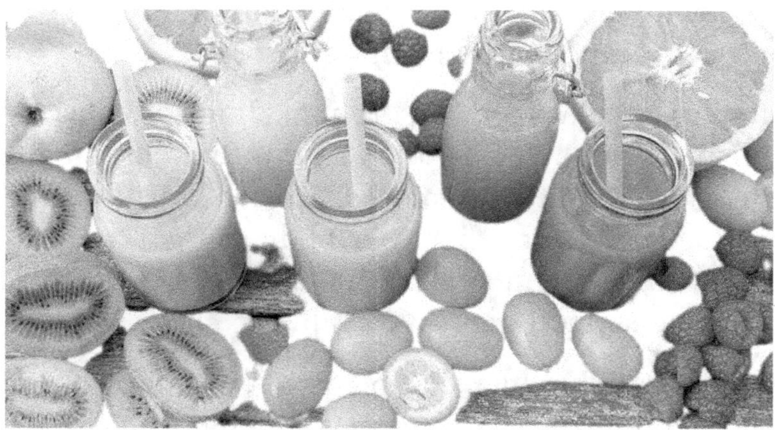

CHAPTER 2

Benefits of Juicing for Gut Health

Juicing has become increasingly popular as a way to improve gut health. The nutrients found in fruits and vegetables are essential for maintaining a healthy digestive system. Here are some of the benefits of juicing for gut health:

Improved Nutrient Absorption: Juicing helps to break down the cell walls of fruits and vegetables, making the nutrients more easily absorbed by the body. This means that your body can get more of the vitamins, minerals, and antioxidants that it needs to support digestive health.

Increased Fiber Intake: Fiber is an essential nutrient that supports healthy digestion and regulates bowel movements. Juicing can provide a concentrated source of fiber, which can help to promote regularity and reduce constipation.

Improved Digestive Function: Juicing can help to improve digestive function by supporting the growth of beneficial gut bacteria. The nutrients found in fruits and vegetables help to nourish the cells that line the gut and support the growth of beneficial bacteria, which are critical for optimal digestive health.

Reduced Inflammation: Chronic inflammation in the gut is a common cause of digestive issues. Juicing can help to reduce inflammation by providing a concentrated source of anti-inflammatory compounds, such as ginger and turmeric.

Boosted Immune System: The gut is home to a significant portion of the immune system. Juicing can help to support immune function by providing a concentrated source of vitamins and minerals that are essential for immune health.

Weight Loss: Juicing can be an effective way to support weight loss by providing a low-calorie, nutrient-dense source of food. The fiber found in fruits and vegetables can help to promote feelings of fullness, which can reduce overall calorie intake and support weight loss.

In conclusion, juicing for gut health can provide a range of benefits, from improved nutrient absorption and digestive function to reduced inflammation and boosted immune function. By incorporating a variety of fruits and vegetables into your juicing routine, you can support the health of your gut and promote overall wellbeing.

CHAPTER 3

Juicing Recipes for Gut Health

Juicing for gut health is an effective way to support digestive function and promote overall wellbeing. Here are some delicious and nutritious juicing recipes that are specifically designed to support gut health:

Green Juice Recipe:

Ingredients:

1 cucumber

2 celery stalks

1 green apple

1 lemon

1-inch piece of ginger

Handful of spinach

Handful of parsley

Directions:

Wash all the ingredients.

Peel the lemon and ginger.

Cut the cucumber, celery, and apple into smaller pieces.

Add all the ingredients to the juicer.

Serve and enjoy!

This green juice recipe is packed with nutrients that are essential for gut health. The cucumber and celery provide a concentrated source of water, which helps to hydrate the body and support digestion.

The green apple adds a touch of sweetness while providing fiber, which supports healthy bowel movements. The lemon and ginger provide anti-inflammatory compounds that can help to soothe the digestive system.

Beet and Carrot Juice Recipe:

Ingredients:

1 medium-sized beetroot

2 carrots

1 green apple

1-inch piece of ginger

Directions:

Wash all the ingredients.

Peel the beetroot, ginger, and carrots.

Cut the ingredients into smaller pieces.

Add all the ingredients to the juicer.

Serve and enjoy!

This beet and carrot juice recipe is a great way to support gut health. Beetroots are rich in nitrates, which help to improve blood flow to the digestive system, supporting healthy digestion. Carrots provide a concentrated source of fiber, which promotes regular bowel movements.

The green apple adds a touch of sweetness while providing vitamin C, which supports immune function. Ginger provides anti-inflammatory compounds that can help to reduce inflammation in the gut.

Pineapple and Papaya Juice Recipe:

Ingredients:

1 cup of chopped pineapple

1 cup of chopped papaya

1 lime

1-inch piece of ginger

Directions:

Wash all the ingredients.

Peel the ginger and lime.

Cut the pineapple and papaya into smaller pieces.

Add all the ingredients to the juicer.

Serve and enjoy!

This pineapple and papaya juice recipe is a delicious way to support gut health. Pineapple and papaya contain enzymes, such as bromelain and papain, which help to break down food and support digestion. The lime provides a concentrated source of vitamin C, which supports immune function. Ginger provides anti-inflammatory compounds that can help to soothe the digestive system.

In conclusion, juicing for gut health is an effective way to support digestive function and promote overall wellbeing. By incorporating these delicious and nutritious juicing recipes into your daily routine, you can provide your body with the essential nutrients it needs to maintain a healthy gut. So why not give it a try and see how juicing can benefit your gut health and overall wellbeing!

Smoothie Bowl

Smoothie bowls have become a popular breakfast or snack option, particularly among health-conscious individuals. A smoothie bowl is essentially a thicker version of a smoothie that is served in a bowl and topped with various toppings. Here are some of the key elements of a smoothie bowl:

Base:

The base of a smoothie bowl is typically a blend of fruits and vegetables that have been frozen to create a thick and creamy texture. Common ingredients include bananas, berries, mango, and spinach. The base is often sweetened with a natural sweetener, such as honey, maple syrup, or dates.

Liquid:

To blend the base, a liquid is added. The liquid can be anything from water to plant-based milk, coconut water, or yogurt. The liquid helps to create the right consistency for the smoothie bowl.

Toppings:

The toppings for a smoothie bowl can be anything from fresh fruit to nuts, seeds, granola, or shredded coconut. The toppings add texture and flavor to the smoothie bowl and make it a more satisfying meal.

Benefits of Smoothie Bowls:

Smoothie bowls are a great way to pack in a variety of nutrients in one meal. The fruits and vegetables used in the base provide essential vitamins, minerals, and antioxidants, while the toppings can add protein, healthy fats, and fiber. Smoothie bowls are also a great way to support digestive health, as they can be customized with ingredients that are specifically targeted at improving gut health. Plus, they're an easy and delicious way to incorporate more fruits and vegetables into your diet.

Tips for Making a Delicious Smoothie Bowl:

Use frozen fruit to create a thick and creamy texture.

Add a liquid slowly to ensure the right consistency for the smoothie bowl.

Experiment with different flavor combinations, such as adding herbs like mint or basil, or spices like cinnamon or ginger.

Use toppings that add texture and flavor, such as fresh fruit, nuts, seeds, or granola.

If you want to add more protein to your smoothie bowl, consider adding a scoop of protein powder or Greek yogurt.

In conclusion, smoothie bowls are a delicious and nutritious way to start your day or enjoy as a snack. They're easy to customize with a variety of fruits and vegetables, and can be topped with anything from nuts to granola. So why not try making a smoothie bowl at home and discover the delicious and nutritious benefits for yourself!

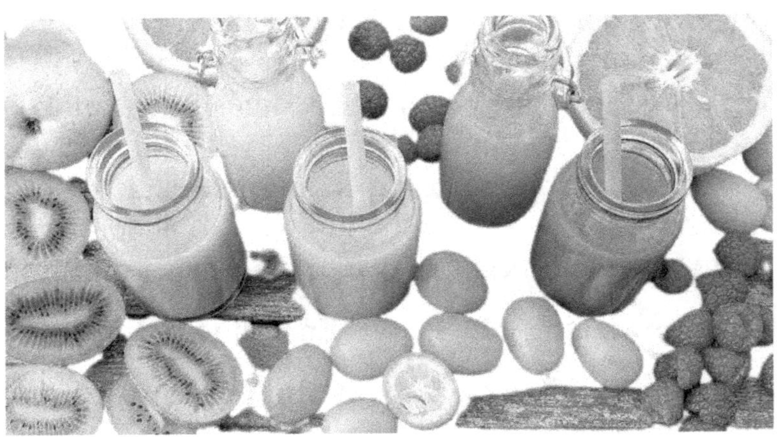

Green Juice

Green juice is a type of juice that is made primarily with green vegetables and fruits. It has become increasingly popular in recent years due to its many health benefits. Here are some of the key elements of green juice:

Ingredients:

Green juice typically includes a combination of green vegetables such as kale, spinach, celery, cucumber, and parsley. These are often combined with fruits such as apples, pears, and citrus fruits to add a touch of sweetness and balance out the bitterness of the vegetables. Some people also add herbs like ginger or turmeric for added flavor and health benefits.

Benefits:

Green juice is a great way to pack in a variety of nutrients in one drink. The vegetables used in green juice are rich in essential vitamins, minerals, and antioxidants, while the fruit adds natural sweetness and fiber. Green juice is also a great way to support digestive health, as it can be customized with ingredients that are specifically targeted at improving gut health. Additionally, green juice is an easy and delicious way to incorporate more vegetables into your diet, especially for those who struggle to eat enough vegetables in their regular meals.

Tips for Making Delicious Green Juice:

Start with a good quality juicer - this can make all the difference in the taste and texture of your green juice.

Use fresh, organic vegetables and fruits whenever possible to ensure the best taste and nutrient content.

Experiment with different flavor combinations - try adding ginger or turmeric for added health benefits or citrus fruits for a tangy taste.

If you find the taste too bitter, start with a smaller amount of greens and gradually increase as your taste buds adjust.

Drink green juice immediately after making it to get the most nutrients and freshest taste.

In conclusion, green juice is a delicious and nutritious way to incorporate more vegetables into your diet. It is packed with essential vitamins, minerals, and antioxidants, and can be customized with ingredients that are specifically targeted at improving gut health. With a good quality juicer and fresh, organic ingredients, anyone can enjoy the delicious and healthful benefits of green juice.

Vegetable Juice

Vegetable juice is a type of juice that is made primarily from a variety of fresh vegetables. Vegetable juice has become increasingly popular in recent years as people are looking for ways to incorporate more vegetables into their diet. Here are some of the key elements of vegetable juice:

Ingredients:

Vegetable juice typically includes a combination of vegetables such as carrots, celery, beets, cucumbers, spinach, kale, and bell peppers. Some people also add herbs like parsley or cilantro for added flavor and health benefits.

Benefits:

Vegetable juice is a great way to pack in a variety of nutrients in one drink. The vegetables used in vegetable juice are rich in essential vitamins, minerals, and antioxidants, and can help boost the immune system, improve digestion, and support overall health. Additionally, vegetable juice is an easy and delicious way to incorporate more vegetables into your diet, especially for those who struggle to eat enough vegetables in their regular meals.

Tips for Making Delicious Vegetable Juice:

Start with fresh, organic vegetables whenever possible to ensure the best taste and nutrient content.

Use a good quality juicer - this can make all the difference in the taste and texture of your vegetable juice.

Experiment with different flavor combinations - try adding a touch of lemon or ginger for added flavor and health benefits.

Drink vegetable juice immediately after making it to get the most nutrients and freshest taste.

If you find the taste too bitter, start with a smaller amount of vegetables and gradually increase as your taste buds adjust.

In conclusion, vegetable juice is a delicious and nutritious way to incorporate more vegetables into your diet. It is packed with essential vitamins, minerals, and antioxidants, and can help boost the immune system, improve digestion, and support overall health. With a good quality juicer and fresh, organic ingredients, anyone can enjoy the delicious and healthful benefits of vegetable juice.

Fruit Juice

Fruit juice is a type of juice that is made primarily from a variety of fresh fruits. It is a popular and refreshing beverage that is enjoyed by people of all ages around the world. Here are some of the key elements of fruit juice:

Ingredients:

Fruit juice typically includes a combination of fruits such as oranges, apples, pineapples, grapes, and berries. Some people also add other fruits such as mangoes, papayas, and bananas for added flavor and health benefits.

Benefits:

Fruit juice is a great way to pack in a variety of nutrients in one drink. The fruits used in fruit juice are rich in essential vitamins, minerals, and antioxidants, and can help boost the immune system, improve digestion, and support overall health. Additionally, fruit juice is a delicious way to incorporate more fruit into your diet, especially for those who struggle to eat enough fruit in their regular meals.

Tips for Making Delicious Fruit Juice:

Start with fresh, ripe fruits whenever possible to ensure the best taste and nutrient content.

Use a good quality juicer or blender - this can make all the difference in the taste and texture of your fruit juice.

Experiment with different flavor combinations - try adding a touch of ginger or mint for added flavor and health benefits.

Drink fruit juice immediately after making it to get the most nutrients and freshest taste.

If you want to reduce the sugar content of your fruit juice, try adding some vegetables such as carrots or beets to balance out the sweetness.

In conclusion, fruit juice is a delicious and nutritious way to incorporate more fruit into your diet. It is packed with essential vitamins, minerals, and antioxidants, and can help boost the immune system, improve digestion, and support overall health. With a good quality juicer or blender and fresh, ripe fruits, anyone can enjoy the delicious and healthful benefits of fruit juice. However, it is important to consume fruit juice in moderation as it can be high in sugar and calories.

It's worth noting that not all fruit juices are created equal. Some commercially available fruit juices are heavily processed and contain added sugars, preservatives, and artificial flavors. These types of fruit juices can be high in calories and may not offer the same health benefits as fresh, homemade fruit juice. To ensure that you are getting the most nutritional value from your fruit juice, it's important to choose whole, fresh fruits and to make your own juice at home whenever possible.

Another consideration is that fruit juice lacks the fiber that is found in whole fruits. Fiber is an essential component of a healthy diet, as it helps to regulate digestion, control blood sugar levels, and reduce the risk of chronic diseases such as heart disease and diabetes. While fruit juice can still be a healthy part of your diet, it's important to also consume whole fruits to ensure that you are getting the full range of health benefits that fruits offer.

Overall, fruit juice can be a delicious and healthful way to incorporate more fruit into your diet. By choosing fresh, ripe fruits and making your own juice at home, you can enjoy all of the nutritional benefits that fruit has to offer. Just remember to consume fruit juice in moderation and to also include whole fruits and vegetables in your diet for optimal health.

CONCLUSION

In conclusion, juicing can be an excellent way to promote gut health and overall wellness. By incorporating nutrient-dense fruits, vegetables, and other ingredients into your juicing recipes, you can support your digestive system, improve your immune function, and boost your energy levels.

Whether you prefer a green juice packed with leafy greens or a sweet and tangy fruit juice, there are endless possibilities when it comes to juicing for gut health. With a little creativity and experimentation, you can find the perfect juicing recipes to suit your taste preferences and health goals.

Remember that juicing should not replace a healthy, balanced diet, but rather complement it. It is important to consume a variety of whole foods, including fruits, vegetables, whole grains, lean proteins, and healthy fats, to ensure that you are getting all of the essential nutrients that your body needs.

By incorporating juicing into a healthy lifestyle, you can support your digestive health, increase your energy and vitality, and feel your best. So go ahead and give juicing a try - your gut will thank you for it!